SIMPLY MAMA FEARLESS

A One-Day Read (Seriously)

By Elizabeth Jimenez
Author and Creator of MamaFearless.com

*Encouragement and Inspiration
for the Amazing Mama-To-Be*

*For God hath not given us a
spirit of fear;but of power, and
of love, and of a sound mind.*

II Timothy 1:7

Introduction

Hello, Mama-to be. First of all, congratulations on your beautiful, wonderful pregnancy! You have all the support of Mama Fearless behind you, as well as my personal prayer for your journey. There is nothing more beautiful than bringing life into this world, and your experience deserves to be one of courage, adaptability, and joy.

All too often we find ourselves inundated with negative influences that are counterproductive to our pregnancy and childbirth experiences. Whatever the motivation, these influences can cause us to doubt our own abilities and even grow fearful of the process—as if we need more apprehension, right?

Simply Mama Fearless is created for mamas by a mama who experienced all of the above and had to learn what it means to give birth fearlessly—through hitches, glitches and all the good and bad in between.

I hope that you enjoy this (short) read, and that you feel inspired, encouraged and confident by the time you reach the end. It won't take you long to read this—I understand all too well how hard it is to fit a lengthy book into a busy, nauseated pregnancy. I spared all the excess, as well as the onslaught of medical advice that you don't really need from me.

Instead, I want you to understand that you have support, you have a cheerleader, and you have a friend in Simply Mama Fearless.

Love and prayers,

Elizabeth

CONTENTS

1. THE WAR CHAPTER

Scared to death. Inadequate. Excited. Motivated. Fascinated. Stupefied. Awed. Terrified.

Just so you know you're not alone. I felt all of the above, too. Getting my pregnancy confirmed was one of the most incredible moments of my life. I say incredible because of the onslaught of completely opposing emotions that overtook me in seconds.

My pregnancy journey was a ten-month road of revelations. Obviously, it was the crazy adventure pregnancy is supposed to be because of, well, pregnancy. But I also found myself in a war zone. I know I'm not the only woman out there who found herself in this position. I got the exciting news of my pregnancy, and then came all the *advice*.

My, oh my. If I could tell you all the advice I received. It's laughable. But beyond all that, I started to feel pulled in two directions. One was that I needed to see a doctor immediately. I needed the doctor to tell me what do so I didn't hurt my baby. The other, stay out of the doctor's office or I'd wind up with a c-section and a host of interventions that would hurt me and my baby.

Now what?

That was the most frustrating part of my entire pregnancy journey, as far as I'm concerned. These weren't just points of view. These were *indoctrinations* of the time we live in. Choosing a side felt something like joining a political party. And both sides left

God completely out of the picture. It also evoked something inside me that I absolutely reviled.

Fear.

Anyone who knows me knows I don't do fear. The normal insecurities and little things that we work through are one thing. But a perpetual feeling of fear of harm or danger? That was *not* happening.

So, I made a little pact with myself. I decided, right out of the gate, that if something made me feel afraid, I was going to wage war against it.

Pregnancy comes with its own little set of fears. These fears are more like insecurities and questions: Am I ready? Can I do this? Does it hurt?

Those questions are normal, and the answers come naturally because you'll work through them.

But being plagued by fear that a doctor is out to get you, or that the doctor is the only way to have a healthy baby is *not* normal. These are fears that have been developed over the last few generations—not throughout womankind.

I decided that I would tap into the instincts that God gave me, the instincts of being a *woman*, who was created with all the necessary things to carry and deliver a child. I didn't need a doctor, midwife, nurse, or doula to tell me that. I didn't need the affirmation of a stranger to remind me I was a woman of God, made in His image.

In today's culture, you will find that pregnancy is viewed as either an illness or proof of the empowered woman. The idea of being a God-created human-being with a soul and given the great commission of the miracle of life is considered outdated, irrelevant and even ignorant by some.

But there is absolutely no denying the deep, spiritual connection I felt during my pregnancy, particularly my labor and delivery. There was such a beautiful connection between my body and my soul and my Creator, awash in a "peace that passes all understanding". No mater what influences out there try to erase the concept of God from life, living and pregnancy, you can't. You just can't.

And God does not give us the spirit of fear. If we feel fear, it's not from God.

This outlook came in handy throughout my entire pregnancy. It started when I was told I wouldn't be able to see a doctor until I was three months along, for very sad and discouraging reasons. Their outlook is basically, "we see too many patients already, and the first three months are fragile. If your pregnancy makes it that long, we'll see you then."

Ouch.

My insurance didn't cover a midwife and I wasn't willing to go into debt to pay for one. Some people make that decision, and that's great, too. I'd had some of the advice of friends' midwives imparted to me, and I actually found myself disagreeing with some of the things I heard.

I prefer a more natural approach to things. However, I am against something that gains credibility by casting suspicion on other. Again, I could feel the fear seeping through. I couldn't be sure if it was the teachings given to these ladies or their own interpretations. Either way, I didn't like feeling like choosing a certain type of medical professional would be viewed as "wrong" by others.

What I'm saying is that your first battle when you become pregnant will most likely be the route you choose to take. You have the freedom to choose whichever road makes you feel comfortable. Be forewarned—you will be pressured. Honest, well-meaning people will urge you in one direction or another based on their experiences and their desire to help. That's really kind of them, but for you, *you* must choose the professional road (or not) that makes you feel like you are on the right path. Pray about it, ask God to deal with you. Go. With. Your. Gut.

I chose a doctor. I worked in the health care industry for nearly a decade and was comfortable with doctors. No, I do not believe that doctors are perfect. Nor do I believe that doctors are out to make the extra buck and are willing to put your safety at risk to do so.

Doctors are highly knowledgeable people in their profession and are paid to offer their medical advice and treatment. They are ultimately paid by you. Sometimes, we feel insecure because we don't know what they know, and sometimes do not understand everything they say. That does not excuse us from being responsible for our own health care and asking questions and making the *ultimate* decision.

Yes, we get to make the ultimate decision. It's your body, and you are completely in control of what you allow a doctor to do. They understand it, too. Some get grouchy when they're delayed or get annoyed with patients asking questions. I've experienced that as well. But that doesn't mean I'm doing anything wrong. That means that they need to be reminded about *informed consent,* and maybe work on their bedside manner.

My first OB doctor made me feel like there wasn't time to ask questions. I gave it two appointments. I did not feel comfortable in the relationship at all. I changed to another OB, and I absolutely loved her.

If you choose a midwife or a doula, you have the same right. In fact, you actually get to interview doulas. After speaking with one and reading the bios on pages of doula websites, I decided against a doula for my own reasons. Midwives and doulas take a more internationally traditional route. They are less likely to use medical interventions than a doctor would. They will also educate you in some aspects of pregnancy that a doctor may not. With a midwife, you will most likely have the option of having your baby at home or a birthing center, if it is safe and low-risk.

You have the right to choose which route you want to take during pregnancy and should never feel guilty about taking it.

When I was unsure of a decision regarding my pregnancy, I prayed about it. I allowed God to direct me through conviction and His voice in prayer.

I had the opportunity to meet with a doula. She asked me a couple questions, asked where I was being seen and about my doctor. Then she fervently stated that I needed to get out of the medical group I was being seen by because they would push me into a c-section. I was told to change my insurance if I could and go to a completely different hospital as well.

What?

She didn't mean anything more than to passionately help. But I felt fear start to bully me. I kindly thanked her for her advice and moved on with my pregnancy, without hiring a doula. I might add that the hospital where I gave birth has a low c-section rate and my OB was a delightful lady. I'm glad I went with my gut.

That is an example of what I am warning you about. It is one thing to have a friendly person offer you their honest advice. But when you start to feel pushed and bullied, stop and evaluate.

Is it your own insecurities about what you know? Is it because someone is being too pushy or attacking your ideas? The person may not be intending to be pushy, but the strong belief system may begin to undermine your confidence.

Not every situation is the same, either. I have a close friend that hired a doula who noticed a glitch during labor in the hospital and helped my friend avoid what would have been a highly likely c-section using traditional methods. Had it not been for the doula, the course of all of my friend's future pregnancies would have been different. She had chosen a doula based on her gut instinct, and that worked out wonderfully for her.

When push comes to shove, *you* are the mama. Tap into the mama instinct that God gave you.

Doctor, nurse, midwife, doula, friend, relative, neighbor, store cashier… whomever. It doesn't matter. They aren't carrying your baby.

Go with your gut.

2. THE UNTHINKABLE CHAPTER

So we just stepped right on the soft spot that people tip-toe around. We just walked all over doctors, doulas, mid-wives, and so on. Since I'm already in this deep, I'll go a step further.

Once the news of my pregnancy was out there, I was given books from all over the place. I was also recommended book titles and I purchased some of my own. I had a lovely pillar of pregnancy books on my nightstand—enough to nearly fend me off from writing this one.

I spent the end of each day in bed with my tea, reading about pregnancy. That phase lasted for all of about two weeks. My cute little idea of reading and tea came to a screeching halt when I noticed a running theme through several of the books.

Let me put it this way. After the first three days of reading, I raced to the nearest whole foods-type store and spent hundreds —yes, *hundreds*—of dollars on all organic, natural foods, body and hair care, and household products. I was in a flurry of fear that everything in my environment was toxic and would hurt my baby.

The anxiety that I felt was tremendous and began influencing me down a path I didn't even realize I was taking. I even found myself questioning the decisions I'd made up to this point.

Had I done the right thing?

When I felt that fear, I remembered my little pact. I was not going to be bullied by the feelings of fear and anxiety that seemed to come from the most unexpected places.

I did the unthinkable.

I closed the books. All of them. Some of them had some helpful ideas, but I didn't want to wade through the pages of scary stuff or fear-motivated stuff to find it. If I had a specific question, I'd set about finding the answer to that one question in whatever way I chose. A lot of times it was online. A lot of times I asked women who'd had babies and who had a positive, Christian outlook.

I decided that too much information was actually working against me. Yes, I wanted to know about how a baby develops and what to expect during the birth. I wanted to know the best way to take care of and protect my pregnancy. The difference was that I was going to control and censor the amount of information I internalized as I found it.

Let's just set it all aside and look at things in a basic light. Do we really need to understand all the possible birth defects to know the importance of a healthy diet? If we're honest, we can most likely say that as soon as we saw the positive line on the home pregnancy test, we were already making decisions to change our lifestyle.

Why is that?

It's because you knew that you were going to be a mama. You knew that you were going to carry a child, and this baby was going to depend on you for everything. That concept *immediately* became the foundation of the decisions you made. That doesn't mean you understood everything about pregnancy or that you knew all the medical information you needed to. But what it *does* mean is that you were *aware*. That's the start.

There's no replacement for a good dose of common sense. Mix that in with your mama instinct and some prayer and you'll feel a whole lot better. You won't need to read about someone else's terrible birth experience to know that.

So why add the anxiety? If you can read through the books and filter out all the fear, then more power to you. There are a lot of healthy tips and fun facts to enjoy. But, if the inundation of knowledge brings you to a place of fear, insecurity and indecision, stop and evaluate.

Every single pregnancy journey is different. It's one path taken by millions of women, but each step is tailor-made. There are things you will do that others may or may not have done. That's why being pushed down a certain path or feeling pressured to take specific steps is a warning sign to you.

A health care professional is there to *advise.* Friends are there to *support* and *listen.* Confidants are there to *provide feedback.* But the rest of your journey is personal. Your baby is being carried by *you.*

You will not hear me direct you down any path or push you to take certain steps. But you will hear me fight for you.

I will fight against fear and anxiety. I will tell you, with every ounce of influence I have, to do whatever it takes to defeat fear. Fear, anxiety and worry will drown out the voice of God. It will strip you of your confidence to make decisions. It will cause you to place the responsibility of your child into someone else's hands.

The moment you begin to doubt your ability to be pregnant, to carry a child and bring it into this world, stop and evaluate. What is causing this? Is it coming from inside of you? If so, then you can deal with yourself and overcome it. But is the doubt being planted from an outside source?

It has become a marketable idea. People everywhere make money from the concept that you cannot give birth properly without the help of ____________ (insert product or service here). It's profitable to cause doubt, to cause you to say, "I must have this or do this in order to successfully have my baby."

As a result, we become insecure, doubtful of our own ability, and then we spend money on whatever it is that we feel we need. Honestly, that's a marketing tool of the day, and it's used on pretty much everything. "I cannot properly mop my floor unless

I use _______", or "I'm not getting the nutrition I need unless I switch my brand of peanut butter to _______"

There is a difference in an internal belief system and feeling influenced by another idea. I encountered this influence while I was pregnant, and with all the hormones, emotions, exhaustion, and nausea, I was particularly gullible. It made me feel insecure, inadequate and ignorant.

But I also discovered that I felt *much* more comfortable and capable after conversations with positive, experienced mothers. They were happy, secure, and helpful. They'd been down that road, had conquered their own set of fears, believed in pregnancy, and believed in me. I didn't agree with everything they all said, but I didn't have to. I just enjoyed being around them. They were phenomenal women.

My mother is one of them. She was perhaps one of the most unknowledgeable women I spoke with when it came to all the new, medical facts we know about pregnancy today. It has been, after all, over twenty-five years since she gave birth to her youngest child. But she was one of the wisest, most incredible sources of *instinctive* and *spiritual* knowledge I ever found. Not because she's my mother, but because she's gutsy. She's tapped into that "mama thing" and doesn't doubt it.

And she didn't buy into every new idea, even when I did.

It took me spending way too much money on things that, in complete honesty, made no difference in my pregnancy and birth experience in order to realize that we don't have to buy in to every idea that's out there, no matter how popular.

It also solidified that fact that there is *no* substitute on this earth for that mama instinct. For me, that meant ousting all the pregnancy books.

Go. With. Your. Gut.

3. THE "ROLL WITH IT" CHAPTER

I learned something else that was very valuable on my pregnancy journey. It's also something I've observed many times over in other women's journeys.

It is the most natural thing to get a plan cemented in place. *This is how I will be pregnant, this is what I will do, and this is exactly how I will have my baby.*

While it's great to be motivated and set goals, it's so easy to forget one big factor in our planning—real life.

My plan was to be practically perfectly pregnant in every way. I was going to exercise, eat right, gain the bare minimum amount of weight, and breeze through those nine-plus months.

Ha!

I craved cheeseburger sliders, fish sticks and strawberry shakes.

I also encountered back trouble at the end of my first trimester.

The day I discovered my back pain was a shocking disappointment. I went to church and rode happily home. When I got out of the car, I couldn't stand upright, and I couldn't walk. My husband had to carry me into the house. After an hour of using a heating pad, ice packs, and resting, I was able to shuffle to the bedroom and flop into bed. The next morning, I was fine.

Okaaaay, so what was that?

My OB didn't seem overly concerned by the problem. While it was rather early for sciatica, back problems are common during pregnancy. There wasn't much I could do to find a diagnosis, as imaging is considered high-risk during pregnancy.

As weeks went by, my back problems intensified. If I was on my feet for hours, I couldn't stand back up once I sat down. My primary doctor suspected a couple possible conditions, but of course there was no confirming anything without imaging.

I was referred to physical therapy and written off work. My job in the health care industry was highly fast-paced and consisted of me being almost entirely on my feet. There was no way I could continue working as planned with this condition. I loved my job and the doctor I worked for, and it was disappointing to have to leave so soon. It was also a complete change of plans. I had been quite set on working up until just before my due date.

I started walking for one to two hours every day, with stretches and exercises. My husband went with me, and we trekked all over our hilly neighborhood. The walking and combined exercises helped, along with the physical therapy, but my bump was growing—fast. It became apparent as time went by that walking was not going to work. I was slowing down and my back was starting to scream at me again.

This was another disappointment. I was used to walking miles' worth of steps at work and having to slow down was difficult for me. I instinctively avoided sitting on the couch, vegging out. I knew in my gut that would work against my labor and delivery. Yes, I know it's commonly expressed that staying active is important to a healthy pregnancy. But I had pushed all of that away. I was following my mama instinct.

I remember standing at the kitchen sink, staring out at our empty pool. Something in me yearned to be in that pool so badly I felt the tears well up. That's not like me. Even though pregnancy can sometimes make you feel like you're not quite yourself, that deep surge of emotion was more than a hormonal moment. I knew I had to follow it.

My husband set about preparing and filling up the pool. I was out there in my straw hat and flip flops, helping in whatever way I could. I was so excited when the water came on and began filling up the pool. I sat on the steps and waited.

It was late February-early March in Southern California. That meant it varied from anywhere between sixty to seventy-five degrees. If the sun was out, I was in that pool. My husband surprised me with a nice quality floating raft with a cup holder. I'd exercise and swim for a while, and then I'd lay on my raft with my fizzy water and straw hat, and just let the sun and the rhythmic motion of the water soothe me to a nap.

That turned my pregnancy journey around. The physical therapy was okay, but it wasn't cutting it. The birthing ball exercises were okay, but again, weren't cutting it. But swimming made all the difference.

My back was still troublesome, but now I was able to exercise and relax at the same time. It didn't hurt that I was always hot and couldn't seem to cool down. I remember my husband shaking his head, wearing a hoodie and jeans, while I happily flopped into the pool.

This little story from my journey is a prime example that things *will* happen during pregnancy, things that we don't exactly count on. You'll hear it said that pregnancy is rarely ever black and white. There are a lot of gray zones. I found this to be true.

For my type-A, systematic and routine-oriented personality, this was a difficult concept to accept. Having to be willing to go with the flow and accept plan changes was perhaps one of the biggest mental challenges I faced. Once I learned how to cope, my stress level decreased considerably.

I relied on that feeling, that *something* that caused my not-really-a-cry-person self to nearly break down at the sight of the empty pool. It was that *something* that drew me to the pool, to swimming, and ultimately salvaged my pregnancy experience. Believe me, the pain was excruciating and had it not been for the pool I would have been pregnant in misery.

I was learning, as will you, to go with my gut.

4. THE IMAGE CHAPTER

We've all seen those pictures online, on the covers of books, of these beautiful women who look as though the only place they've changed during pregnancy is in their tummies—and that's not until they're at least six months along.

Well, I've seen women like that. I wasn't one of them. I was one of the "are you *sure* you aren't having twins?" women. Yeah. I got it from everywhere. By the end of my first trimester there was a bump. By the middle of my second trimester I was quite clearly pregnant.

I'm about five feet tall. I'm as high-waisted as they come. There was nowhere to go but out. And, I'll be completely upfront in saying that I indulged in the few cravings I had. I didn't go crazy, neither was always the most disciplined pregnant person.

When it comes to pregnancy, we are all so different, and we'll carry our babies differently. You'll get all the predictions of whether or not you're having a boy or girl based on how you gain. You'll get comparisons of so-and-so's daughter and how they gained compared to you. You'll get comments from the peanut gallery. I even had a few men comment on my bump.

By the time all the comments were rolling in, I had been forced to adapt to so many other things that all I could do was laugh. It would have been easy to get hurt about the freedom people felt to comment on my progress, but I just didn't have the energy to deal with it. I simply laughed it all off.

I would have people ask how far along I was, look at my belly, and then ask again or repeat my answer back to me in question, as if I'd made a mistake. Surely, I had to be further along!

The really *good* comments came along as I was approaching my June due date. The "you look miserable" ones and the "It's *got* to be soon—you don't look like you can go any longer" comments got richer by the week.

By this time, I was dead tired, my back was almost always aching and pinching, and my emotions were on edge. The comments were now smarting. I never actually cried, but I fought my temper and the urge to make equally unkind comments. It's funny how people, who have absolutely *no* room to talk, will comment on your weight and shape.

I had to remind myself that just because someone was unkind to me didn't make it right to respond in the same manner. I couldn't allow my emotions to get carried away. I know that this sounds a little odd. It is widely stated that when you're pregnant, you have the right to act in any way you feel. My mother, however, didn't raise me that way, and she was now staying with me until I delivered. Just having her near reminded me that I shouldn't give in to my emotions.

You may be wondering why I'm even mentioning this. Well, the answer is because there isn't a lot of professional discussion about the ride your emotions take during pregnancy, and some of the things that make it worse.

For me, it was bizarre to watch my body transform in a matter of months, completely out of my control, and feel the emotional changes that went with it. My husband was supportive and loving through every part of the journey (bless him), but that didn't necessarily cure me of the challenges I faced internally.

I had to seriously question the integrity of my belief system and self-image. Did I *really* believe that I was God's creation, and beautiful in His sight, or was that ingrained rhetoric? Did I honestly believe my husband when he told me I was beautiful?

How *did* I feel about my changing body? What about that funny line that had appeared, or the fact I couldn't even fit my arms into most of my blouses?

There comes a time in our pregnancy when we will all have to face the challenge of self-image. It isn't always easy when you have people making unkind remarks, or when you don't recognize yourself from the neck down. But this is where our true values shine through. I had my husband, my mother, and closest friends encouraging me, telling me that I was carrying a child, and that is a beautiful thing. It was up to me to buy into the true beauty of pregnancy or fall into the world of comparisons and competition.

To be honest, it takes up *way* too much energy to get caught up trying to look perfect by the world's standards. You will save yourself so much trouble if you embrace the new, pregnant you. I allowed myself to be okay with a really (*really*) round tummy and gave up the idea of trying to prove I hadn't doubled in size everywhere else. Instead, I found clothes that were comfortable, laid over my bump and didn't hug the rest of me. I looked bigger because I *was* bigger, but that was okay because I was bringing a child into the world. My priority wasn't to look like a beauty queen. My priority was to accomplish something—doing my part in the miracle of life.

That was how I was able to withstand all the remarks. I saw pictures of women who had pregnant bumps and looked like a slim person who'd swallowed a watermelon seed, and I was genuinely happy for them. I felt wistful at times, wishing I could have been the same. But it wasn't that way, and so I made up my mind not to allow myself to journey down that road. I was having a son, but what if it were a daughter? What would I have wanted her to see from me? What example would I set?

I was so thankful to have the moral support around me to help me come to that conclusion, with the help of the Lord. I want now to share that with you, dear reader. Just know, that when it comes to bearing a child, there is a beauty that cannot be taken away. It doesn't matter how the world views image (clearly it isn't the healthiest as it's currently a major crisis), or how others view you. Focus on your health, and just know that you are amazing.

Maybe this chapter will help you identify when you start feeling insecure and down on yourself, and help you stop and evaluate. Where are the insecurities coming from? What can you do to fend them off?

Go with your gut. And know you're beautiful.

5. THE HUSBAND CHAPTER

I took a moment to ask my husband some questions about our pregnancy journey. The reason for this is because another thing I noticed about pregnancy books, websites and other platforms is that there just isn't a lot out there about the man's perspective. I will be honest and tell you I was pleasantly surprised at the level of response I received. It was a fun conversation to have.

To give you some background, my husband has always been very involved in things taking place in my life. He is extremely family oriented and openly affectionate. He is just geared that way. Before I go into any more details, I want to gently remind you that every husband is different. They don't all fit into the same box. The best way to read this chapter is to use it as more of an open guide of ideas and be willing to adjust it to better fit your spouse's personality.

I learned that Adam, my husband, took this pregnancy seriously. Okay, so that sounds rather obvious. But when I say he took it seriously, he took it seriously as a man. That meant that the result of bringing a child into the world translated into the responsibilities it would bring from here on out. Adam started his own business from the ground up, and we are still in the trenches of growing it. Even with this, Adam had openly communicated his wishes that I stay home to raise our child.

I was not surprised at this (we had discussed it before our marriage) and was happy and excited to do it. We knew that my giving up my job would be a financial sacrifice, but we were willing to make it. We set plans in place to prepare for this new change.

It sounded like were in total control, right?

Wrong.

Adam quickly learned that an enormous part of the pregnancy journey was taking place inside of me, and me only. It was difficult at first for him to find his place. After all, I was the one throwing up, exhausted, growing, required to be at the appointments, and so much more. Where did that leave him?

Determined to be apart, that left him holding my hair back as I lost my meal, driving all over town to multiple restaurants to pick up one dish or another to create the only dinner that sounded appealing to me (I believe the record was dishes from three separate places), and picking up a lot of extra chores around the house.

As time went by, he took on the task of putting together all the baby's furniture as it came in, hanging pictures on the walls, and helping me with the heavy tasks around the house.

It was rather tricky. I'm a pretty independent person, and it's safe to say that in the beginning, he hovered—badly. I felt sick and didn't feel like talking. He needed direction. He needed to be apart of this, too, to be apart of the team. Because I felt nauseous and exhausted, I stopped talking, which effectively cut him out of everything.

But as the weeks went by, we began to develop a husband and pregnant wife relationship. I learned to depend on him as I honestly needed to, and he learned to be there for me when I needed him, but to give me the space I needed as well. That *required* communication.

As the due date drew near, Adam had the car serviced, minor repairs completed around the house, and even began tracking the weather. We made a few different trips to the hospital to time the travel distance in preparation for labor.

While he sounds wonderful, this is not a list of his amazingness. If you notice the tasks he took on, you'll see they were things that I, as a pregnant woman, were not thinking about in my nesting craze. They were tasks that he *did* think about and that made him feel *apart.*

Adam was *not* interested in every medical detail of my pregnancy. He was infatuated with the baby kicking through my tummy. He was *not* infatuated with the articles I read, the statistics of pregnancy, every detail of every appointment I went to.

He would call me when the appointment was over or be waiting for me if he wasn't at work and wanted to know if everything was okay. He was easily overwhelmed by too much medical information. Adam is medically savvy, but he simply couldn't relate. He could sympathize, but he couldn't empathize. What honestly mattered to him was that I was okay, the baby was okay, and the appointment went well. He attended the first appointment and all the ultrasounds. Beyond that, he felt more productive and helpful in other areas.

He also was a lot easier on the physical changes of pregnancy than I expected him to be. While I pondered over my everchanging body and had to work through acceptance, Adam affectionately embraced the changes. The pressures I had expected regarding looking a certain way were clearly coming from within myself and not from him.

I had a preconceived idea in my head of the areas to which he would react during my pregnancy and how he would react. I had missed the mark in nearly everything. He was happy to be helpful, excited to watch the changes, not so excited with all the medical details, and focused on his way of preparation.

Looking back, we realized that things went a lot smoother when I didn't expect him to be my pregnant friend. As he put it, he couldn't possibly understand what it's like to be pregnant. He never would, because he'll never be pregnant. What he *did* want was to be apart of the team. It meant he had a different position while still rooting for the same goal.

A lot of my frustration eased when I stopped trying to share every single aspect of my journey with him. I shared those details with my mom, my also-pregnant cousin, and a close confidant. I should say that it wasn't a complete lack of interest on his part. Adam is a natural "fixer". To hear every detail when it was so far beyond his control only added stress.

And, let's just be honest. He wasn't really interested in blogs about "top most helpful nursery items", or "ten things I wish I'd known about pregnancy". What he was interested in was a plan of action: how were we going to handle the labor and delivery? What were we going to take to the hospital? Did we have a backup plan in case something went differently than expected?

By the time our baby boy arrived, we had paved a road that worked for us. I have *definitely* tucked all these experiences away for later and will be pulling them out next time.

While not every spouse is geared the same way, we learned a principle that's worth sharing. First, you can't expect your spouse to handle the pregnancy the same way you will. It just doesn't happen that way. Second, allow your spouse to be apart of the journey. Let him come up with tasks and things that will make him feel apart. It requires a new level of communication and it's not always easy. We certainly weren't perfect. But we didn't give up, and we have some wonderful memories to share.

And don't expect to get it all right. It's okay if you blunder along the way. It just means you're human, and that's a good thing.

6. THE NURSERY CHAPTER

From the moment we knew we were ready for a baby, I was flipping through photos of different nursery ideas. I had a vision in my head for either a boy or a girl, and I reveled in the idea of creating the perfect nursery.

Then I found out I was pregnant. I was over the moon. The excitement blurred all the days together. I focused on cute ways to share the news. My saved nursery ideas were on my mind, but I didn't worry about them. After all, I was only a few weeks along.

Then the exhaustion hit. I would get up at 6:00 am, be at work by 7:30, be home by 5:00 pm, and crash. And then the nausea hit. I'd get through my work day (throwing up), come home and try to keep some dinner down (throwing up), shower (throwing up), and crash.

Nursery? Yeah, right.

The second bedroom, the one that would be our baby's room, was currently being used as a guest bedroom. The carpet was old and worn out and the room *badly* needed repainting. There was a lot to do. By the time I was three months along, I hadn't purchased a single nursery item. I remember seeing all the cute nursery photos out there and feeling like a complete loser.

Then I got mad.

Who was I kidding? The baby wouldn't even *need* a nursery,

technically, until he was months older. So, what was my true motivation? After some reflection, I realized that, in my own way, I was getting caught up in comparisons. I had given in to the pressure that the nursery should be perfect before baby arrived. My type-A personality demanded it.

But, at the rate I was going, it just wasn't going to happen exactly the way I wanted.

So, I let it go. I made a list of the necessities we would need on hand when we brought Baby home. If we are truly honest, the list of actual necessities is rather small.

I felt great by the beginning of my second trimester, even as my back started to give me some problems. I took a trip to visit family and while I was gone, my husband, father-in-law and sister-in-law pulled up the old carpet, refurbished the hardwood flooring, repainted, and replaced the ceiling fan. I was completely out of the house while the chemicals were used and dried, and by the time I came home, the second room was ripe and ready for me to get to work.

I began price shopping and ordering furniture pieces. Adam put them together as they came in. Slowly but surely, the baby's room transformed. Then, as my pregnancy progressed and my back worsened, I was forced to slow down. The essentials, however, were complete.

Some things weren't even completed until after our son, Kai, was born. And, you know what? It was okay. Adam was working a more than full-time schedule with his business, I was trying to manage our home while slowing down, day by day. There just wasn't room to be perfect. I know that many people bring their babies home from the hospital and the nursery is perfectly ready and waiting.

But, sometimes, it just doesn't happen that way.

The truth is that your baby will most likely be in your room at first. Things that you need on hand will be stationed throughout the house. The time you first spend in the nursery is probably going to be minimal.

If I could share one thing with you, it would be to let yourself *enjoy* the nursery-creating process. If you are putting so much pressure on yourself that it becomes an area of stress, it's probably time to stop and evaluate.

Who said the nursery must be perfect before baby arrives? Where is that pressure coming from? There will be time for pictures. There will be years of memories.

If it is imperative to you to have the nursery complete before you give birth, then you'll know the plans you need to make in advance to have that happen. It's funny how we make things work when it really matters to us.

For me, I realized I couldn't do it all. So, I let it go. And that worked for us. It would have placed unneeded stress on Adam to try and have everything perfect by my due date, and we were already adjusting to so much. We were able to relax when we let that pressure go.

No matter what your priorities are, it's possible to fend off the pressure. And it's okay. There is no reason to feel guilty if you can't do everything you planned. It's part of adjusting through pregnancy, and it's great practice for later! Mom life is all about learning to roll with stuff.

Just remember to tap into your mama instincts. If you start feeling like you're drowning, just stop and evaluate. What do you need to do to minimize your stress?

And then... you guessed it... go with your gut.

7. THE BIRTH PLAN CHAPTER

This one is funny. Plan your birth? Right.

I say this because I was very diligent in researching for a birth plan. And I used none of it. I'll explain that later.

Basically, a birth plan is an organized and written plan of your wishes during your birth experience. It can include labor, delivery, and postpartum care.

Birth plans have become popular in recent years, especially during the rise of the "natural birth" movement. If you were to go online and search out "birth plan", you'd find a whole host of sites and resources to help you. You can also find templates to get you started.

A lot of birth plans focus on things that are considered interventions. Examples of this are: the use of Pitocin, Epidural (and other forms of pain management), the practice of Episiotomy.

Other aspects of labor and delivery planning are: birthing positions, baby monitoring, ability to move around during labor, etc.

Postpartum planning may include things like: delayed cord clamping, administering erythromycin eye ointment to your baby, skin-to-skin, your infant's first immunizations, bottle feeding versus nursing, etc.

Birth planning can be as in-depth as you want it to be. It's your birth experience, so you can get online, research every single facet of the birthing process and put stipulations on each one if you so desire.

Okay—down to real talk.

The use of birth plans has skyrocketed since the publication of certain books and the uprising of the "natural birth" movement. From the moment I announced that I was expecting, I was asked, "are you going natural?"

Well, what exactly does that mean? To some, a natural birth means no Epidural. To others, it means having your babies at home. I learned this by asking many mamas out there and researching throughout my pregnancy. They all had their own answers, based on their own foundation of knowledge. Some had read popular books. Others were following their midwives' advice and quoting their facts. Others had spent time online and in forums.

I believe in having a say in your medical care. Not only is it the responsible thing to do, it's *legal.* It is your moral responsibility to make sure you are informed about your medical care just as much as it's your health care professional's legal responsibility.

However, unless you go to medical school, there are some things you are not going to be able understand well enough to make all the decisions on your own. That is the most basic, real answer you're ever going to hear. I can hear the "all natural" authors and figures throwing this book against the wall.

Yes, it's your own body. Yes, it's your own baby. And yes, some doctors have even pushed unnecessary interventions. But it doesn't change the fact that the doctor knows medically more about the hospital process than you do, and that doctors and midwives know more about the details of birthing in general.

We can either resist it or work with it. Because of a lot of the newer, natural-based books out there, a lot of suspicion is raised against OB doctors and surgeons. That is fine if you're planning on not having your baby in the hospital and can guarantee you won't end up there (which, you can't 100% guarantee).

Because most of us "middle-of-the-roaders" choose to have our baby in the hospital, you don't want to turn your doctor into the enemy in your mind.

I began writing my birth plan after researching and looking at birth plan templates. I noticed that many, *many* templates stated things like "no Pitocin", "no Epidural", "no Erythromycin ointment on the baby's eyes", "no Hepatitis B immunization", "Delayed cord clamping".

Before you write any of these things, thoroughly research what they are. I worked in the health care industry, particularly in eye care, for a decade. When I saw that many were declining Erythromycin, I wanted to know their reasons why. The answers varied. What became clear was that most people didn't know what Erythromycin is used for. Only one mama stated that she had a certain allergy to a class of medications and could not use Erythromycin, therefore did not want to risk using it on her newborn in case he had inherited the allergy.

I brought up the idea of my birth plan to my doctor. She smiled patiently and was a lot nicer than I expected her to be about it. She advised that I bring my birth plan in to one of my prenatal appointments, and in her vernacular, "ensure that it is realistic". This wasn't stated with any trace of sarcasm or disrespect. She stated it honestly, truthfully, and directly.

The truth is that as far as the hospital is concerned, when it comes to our health and safety, decisions will be made to protect mama and baby. If you are going to have your baby in the hospital, it is best to understand that there will be some decisions that doctors will advise you to make. You should be aware of this, and you should have a say. If you do not understand what is being presented to you, you need to ask for clarification.

I decided to do more, down home research for my own birth plan. I asked my doctor about Episiotomy. She explained to me that this practice is considered antiquated and is being phased out. I thoroughly researched the practice and the reasoning behind Episiotomy. After speaking with my doctor and hearing her viewpoint as well, I knew I would specify my wishes on my birth plan.

I took a tour of the hospital in which I would give birth. This was the best decision I made as far as planning my birth. I used the information they gave me, my knowledge of the hospital rooms and my options, to prepare for birth. I also learned that (contrary to what a lot of books generalize about hospitals), my hospital has a low c-section rate. They also do not promote administering Epidural. You can most certainly have one by request, but it is not considered high priority and certainly isn't pushed.

After doing my own research, my birth plan condensed from two pages (typed) to half a page. Most of the things I had originally typed were, in all honesty, redundant. I didn't need to specify skin-to-skin because, if there were no problems, the hospital highly promoted skin-to-skin—and even had case studies to prove the benefits.

The point here is that before you buy into a complete belief system, you need to understand what you're asking. Why are you declining Pitocin (and I did decline with a disclaimer)? Why are you declining Hepatitis B immunization for your infant? Have you cited your sources? Where is your information coming from?

I should also add, that, like myself, some authors of some new, popular books are *not doctors or licensed health care practitioners.* They, like me, are mamas who had their babies and became passionate about certain belief systems.

That is why you will find absolutely no medical advice in this book. What you *will* find is someone fighting for you—fighting against fear and being pressured into any belief system you do not understand or that causes you doubt.

I appreciate the natural birth concept and accredit some good changes in our hospital system to the education being spread by this movement. However, I disagree with any movement or side that casts suspicion on another party. I disagree with doctors scoffing at midwives, or treating their patients like they don't know their own body.

If you wish to be more naturally minded, that is great!

However, if you are planning on having your baby in the hospital, the worst thing you can do is become suspicious of your doctor and distrusting of their decisions. How can you possibly feel safe during your labor and delivery if you become convinced the doctor is trying to make the fast buck or press unnecessary interventions on you?

If you feel that strongly, you may want to consider another route of childbirth. Every mama should feel free to make their decisions based on a clear mind, *free of fear*.

You are the mama. That is your baby. Tap into that fact and understand that there is no other person that can feel your baby the way you can or can understand what is going on inside you to the degree of your own understanding. Doctors are going to make decisions based upon their training and their belief systems, and from what you tell them. Midwives and doulas will coach you and advise you according to their own beliefs as well.

But absolutely *no one* can tell you what to do like you can. Before you make your choices, make sure they are *your* choices. If you choose no Epidural, understand *why* you are choosing no Epidural. If you choose no Erythromycin, understand the medication enough to make an educated decision. And, if you decide to have those things, don't allow anyone to make you feel like a lesser woman or inadequate because you made those decisions.

Finally, allow for the gray zone. I witnessed, over and over, situations where births did not go as planned and interventions were absolutely necessary. Some of these women had set birth plans and were left with emotional guilt and disappointment because things had not gone as they wished. I am not talking about the famous circle of interventions, (Pitocin, Epidural, Pitocin, Cesarean). I am talking about Preeclampsia, needed blood transfusions, and serious conditions that occurred.

The disappointment had drowned out something very beautiful and powerful in these women—they were able to stick it out. They made difficult decisions in order to bring their child into the world. They sacrificed their own ideals and goals to maintain the safety of their baby.

They have beautiful children.

Fear is paralyzing. Fear will cause your instincts to stumble and drown out the internal voice that is so deeply connected to your baby.

Your decisions are your own, and should be made from your own, personal desire—not fear. You are strong enough and capable enough to allow the influence to come from within, not from external sources. There is enough education out there to help you with your choices, but the ultimate decisions are yours alone. There should be no guilt for the path you choose to take.

I personally made the choice to decline Pitocin and Epidural. My reasons were not based upon the influences that are more prominent today. My reason was simply this: I knew that labor was going to be painful. I resolved that I would not be afraid of natural pain. Pain, in labor, does not mean that something is wrong. Labor pain is the most natural pain in existence.

I wanted to feel every part of the process. I wanted to be intimately and spiritually connected to my childbirth, and that meant hurting. God had established that childbirth was a painful process, and I wanted to allow myself this journey in its entirety.

I received comments from people who said, "Give it a few hours and you'll be screaming for an Epidural," and "Don't do that to yourself. Just get the Epidural."

I resolved from the beginning that if I couldn't take it, I'd request an Epidural (if my labor wasn't too advanced for it). I had also made the internal decision that if something happened and I could not deliver naturally, I would make the best decision for my baby, and I would be okay.

I would not allow fear of pain, fear of the process, or *fear of failure* to be present in my childbirth experience.

I waged war against fear.

And I won.

That war, and that victory, set the tone for my delivery.

I believe in you. You can do the same thing. It may mean something different in your experience. It's normal to feel a little fear as the day approaches—especially if it's your first time. It's a big experience. There's a stark difference, however, between a little fear that you can work through and an anxious fear that alters your state of mind.

You can win the war against fear. Believe in yourself. You are the mama. Tap into that protective, mama bear inside you. Hone those instincts.

Go. With. Your. Gut.

8. THE PREPARATION CHAPTER

My June due date was quickly approaching. My date had been moved from the 25th to the 27th but I wasn't paying attention to that. I knew I wasn't going to go that far. I often would state this while conversing, and I had a lot of natural-minded people tell me that I needed to go as long as I could. Forty weeks was the target range of pregnancy.

I nodded politely. I knew I was not going forty weeks. How did I know this? Remember that instinct I've been talking about? Something deep within told me I was not going to make it to June 25th. I was certain of this since my second trimester. I don't know why. Maybe there was something we'll never know about the pregnancy. There are sometimes things we'll just never know. And we don't *have* to know every minute detail.

My mother, a very instinctive person herself, trusted my instincts—sometimes more than I did. She listened when I expressed my feelings and concerns. She encouraged me to follow my gut. She trusted me enough that she even changed all her plans and came from Northern California to stay with us three weeks earlier than she intended. It was a good thing, or she'd have missed the birth.

One of the common struggles first-time mommies face is undermining ourselves. Our instincts will tell us something and we doubt it. Our own insecurities, outside influences, fear, or things we've read will interfere and we'll shut ourselves out of our own pregnancy. This is another reason why I previously stated I stopped reading all those books.

I found myself practicing following that instinctive voice like never before at the end of my pregnancy journey. I had a pre-natal appointment during all this, and afterward I called my dad.

"I just want you to know the doctor told me I'm already dilated to two centimeters. I think you should have your bags packed and ready. I'm not going to go to the 25th."

Being dilated to a 1 or 2 is quite common at the end of preg-nancy. It wasn't being dilated that had me making that call. It was the voice inside that said it was almost time.

I wanted to take maternity photos. I put off scheduling the photo shoot due to being busy, but by the end of May something told me if I didn't get maternity photos taken *now*, there wouldn't be a maternity photo shoot. We managed to get a session in on a hot Memorial Day weekend.

Next came the hospital bag.

I researched necessities from websites and blogs and found so many variances it was overwhelming. From the minimalist to the urban glamor mom, there were options galore. I packed and repacked my bag. At first it was so stuffed I couldn't zip it. I re-evaluated. No, I didn't think my baby would need four outfits, six hats and three pairs of mittens, three pairs of socks, three blan-kets, three burp cloths, two tubes of organic diaper cream, two bottles, ten diapers, a brush, an aspirator and more.

I removed at least half of the items. Now, I could zip my diaper bag.

What I actually ended up using was an even smaller list: One outfit and two hats, one blanket and one burp cloth, and, sometimes, one pair of mittens.

Packing was a fun experience. The excitement of what was to come was contagious.

I was so excited I even created a labor plan, aside from my

birth plan. I had specific music I'd asked my husband to play for me, specific essential oils for aromatherapy, candles, my birthing ball, specific people present, drinks I would like to be offered… you get the idea.

I set my mom and my mom-in-law in charge of making sure all the proper people had my labor and birth plans. A good friend and confidant, Kay, who'd recently given an unmedicated birth was going to assist me in labor, and a plan was formed for transitioning to the hospital.

Because I am very much an introvert, I was determined to labor mostly at home. I didn't want all the hubbub of the hospital interfering with my labor. I didn't want any added stress or pressure. The RN who gave the tour of the hospital had explained the stages of labor and the best time to come into the hospital. She stated that the smoothest labor is done at home, and to wait until contractions were four to five minutes apart, or until my water breaks.

I had decided to wait until transitional labor (the ending stage of labor, just before delivery) before going into the hospital, whether my water broke or not. Because I was choosing to wait to the end, I asked my good friend to be there to help me identify the transitional stage of labor as it came.

I packed a small suitcase for my husband and myself for our hospital stay. I was feeling energetic and a bit restless—and quite moody.

My due date was still two weeks away, but I could feel something changing inside me. My son's birthday was almost here.

It's hard to explain exactly what takes place when you turn the corner and are nearing giving birth. It can be hard to recognize due to the exhaustion and feeling…well…big. Baby is now a good size and is sitting at home right in the middle of you. Balancing, walking, getting out of bed, showering…pretty much everything is a new challenge. Breathing is a chore at times as well. Not that you *can't* breathe, but it just takes more work to get a good breath.

I remember laughing as my husband had to give me a little

push to help me out of bed. I was down to only a couple pairs of shoes that still fit, and only the roomiest of all my maternity outfits were comfortable. Up until this point, I'd been quite proud of the fact that I could still buckle my shoes. Now, I was forced to ask for help. That one was hard for me. I did not relish the days of decreasing independence.

Despite the discomfort of being so stretched and cramped, I was antsy and jittery. I could feel something deep within going off like a sparkler during the 4th of July. It brought even more of a flush to my cheeks (which I did not need). I hustled and bustled about my home, moving this and rearranging that. I made trips to the store to get last minute supplies. My mom, ever patient with me, kept a wary eye as I hobbled down the aisles. My back was a mess and walking was a chore, but I was absolutely determined to accomplish what tasks I could.

This was my last, final spurt of energy in preparation for Baby Boy. This was the last round of nesting to overtake me before the next journey began. I knew it, and so did my mother.

These nine-plus months had taught me something very valuable. I had learned that I was a woman who could adequately carry a child, through hitches and glitches and some extra weight. I was fully able, and I was completely tuned in to the baby inside me. I knew what I felt, that I was *instinctively* aware.

I had learned the skill of going with my gut.

9. MY BIRTH STORY CHAPTER

Wednesday, June 13[th.]

It was a full two weeks before my forty-week due date. But I knew. I was done. Baby was done.

That day I trekked through the store one last time, and though I felt like I was hustling, I *know* I was going at a tortoise's pace. I saw the looks of other shoppers as they watched me in concern. They could see as well as I could, that I was at the end of my pregnancy.

I went to church that night, and I even managed to wear my little, two-inch heels. They were roomy sandals and were one of the only pairs of shoes I had that were still comfortable.

The music started, and I was moving. I was not going to just stand there in discomfort, and I *certainly* was not going to sit in my pew and let the church service pass me by. It was a great service and we all lingered afterward, talking with friends and church family.

Adam, my mother and I were some of the last to leave. I felt tightening in my tummy, but I'd been getting Braxton Hicks for the last two months off and on. While they were becoming more frequent, I wasn't really worried about it.

This was my first pregnancy. I wasn't sure what to expect when it came to contractions. I had spent some time researching things like "what do contractions feel like?" and "what is the difference between Braxton Hicks and actual labor?" After searching for some clear answers, I had to just accept that it wasn't going to be perfectly clear this first time. I was determined not to worry about it, either. I felt in my core that I would just *know.*

That night, standing and chatting after the church service, my tummy became particularly tight. I looked down and watched the tightening through my dress, and figured I was having a contraction. However, I was not going to get wrapped up in the "is this a contraction? Is this it?" questions. I had seen and read enough to know that can drive a mama wild if you let it.

I was craving hot, fast food. I'd tried to curb my unhealthy cravings throughout my pregnancy and was mediocrely successful. But tonight, I was ravenous. We stopped on the way home and I ate enough to feed two grown men. I chuckle now to remember my husband's sideways glances and my mom's "hmm" as I downed the food.

On the way home, I had more tightening. It wasn't painful, but it was tight enough to get my attention. I still wasn't concerned. I had heard so many women talk about their labor experiences, and pain had been a prevalent part of it all. I didn't know what to expect, but I knew it was supposed to hurt—a lot.

We made it home and I got out of the car. More tightening. It was enough that I was unable to walk and was uncomfortable. That was a contraction, I supposed. I hobbled into the house and prepared for bed. I fell fast asleep.

I awoke at 3:00 am on the dot. Something had jolted me out of sleep. I must tell you that I am a very heavy sleeper. I once slept through a Northern California thunder storm—with my windows open. It's a story my family still teases me about to this day.

But on this particular night, whatever awakened me had me *wide* awake and perfectly alert. I hadn't felt anything, but instinctively I was completely aware something was happening in my body.

That's when I felt it. A little popping feeling, sort of like a water balloon gently breaking. I stood up, and it was clear my water had broken. I wasn't sure of what to expect in this area, either. I hurried to the restroom and it was again very, very obvious. My mother was sleeping on her foldaway bed in the nursery, and the door was closed. I hobbled precariously to the door and knocked.

"Yes?" Came a muffled, sleepy voice.

"Can I come in?"

"Yes, just open the door."

Our home is a bungalow built in the 1950's. The doors are still original, and it can require some mild force to twist the knob and open them. As I exerted force to try to open the door, my water continued to break. If this is your first time being pregnant, just be aware that your water breaking isn't always a famous, single *gush*. It can happen in spurts. Well, I learned this while trying to open my mother's door.

"Um, I kind of can't," I finally ended up saying softly through the door.

I heard a frantic ruffle of blankets and the banging of the foldaway bed's legs against our refurbished, hardwood floor. My mom was up and to the door in seconds. The door flew open and she found me standing there, knees together, trying to figure out what to do next.

"My water just broke."

She clasped her hands. "Oh. Oh! Ooooooh!"

The reality of the moment came over us both in that instant. The emotion is indescribable. You will feel it when the certainty of birth finally arrives. It's beautiful, and something beyond words.

"Are you timing your contractions?"

Well, that was just it. I was having tightening, but not any serious pain. I walked into the restroom to tend to my business, and that's when a contraction—an undeniable contraction —hit. It wasn't painful—certainly uncomfortable and I definitely couldn't walk while it lasted.

Looking back, if I had properly identified my contractions, they were about three minutes apart. However, there wasn't serious pain. I kept expecting that ferocious "nothing more painful than contractions" pain to grip me.

I need to stop and say here that I was not afraid. I was a little nervous. There was no helping that, but more than nerves, I felt excitement and anticipation. Fear, however, had been defeated long ago.

I called the nurse advice line connected with my health group. Of course, they advised that since my water had broken, I needed to go to the hospital. They would keep me there until the baby was born.

I hung up and, after tossing ideas back and forth with my mom, I decided I would stay home for just a little while longer to monitor my contractions. I wasn't in any serious pain, after all, and I didn't want to be in the hospital for hours and hours, waiting.

I called my good friend, Kay, who was planning on helping me through my labor. It was now 3:20 am. She, naturally, didn't answer. I left her a voicemail and sent her a text. I figured she would get it soon and would return my call.

I also called my dad in Northern California to alert him of my labor, knowing he would pack up and drive down right away. I wasn't surprised when he didn't answer, either.

Contractions were coming, but they were obscure, not clear enough to time. At 3:30 I woke Adam.

"It's time. My water broke."

He looked at me calmly, then got up, got dressed, and turned on the soft music I had requested. He also called his mother to let her know of my labor. She was at our house in twenty minutes.

I was determined to take time to shower before going to the hospital. Contractions, more noticeable now, came during the shower. Again, not as painful as I had anticipated. It was uncomfortable and incredibly tight feeling, but nothing alarming.

I dressed and braided my hair, experiencing more contractions along the way. Now, I leaned across my birthing ball, letting the rolling motion soothe the tightness. I listened to the soft music playing and just breathed, concentrating on relaxing.

My mom-in-law stepped quietly into the room, watching me. After a few minutes, she nodded and said, "you're going to do just fine, Mama. This is going to be quick."

And with that, she peacefully went into the living room to wait. That soft-spoken affirmation was so empowering.

Things were growing more uncomfortable every few minutes. I went from the birthing ball to the bed where I lay on my side for a while. My mom stood at the side of the bed, massaging my back, offering a quiet presence of support. Adam made himself comfortable on the bed, his feet propped on the birthing ball, and dozed off.

The entire room was calm, dimly lit (which I feel is so important during labor), and completely void of stress or fear.

Then, at 5:30 am, something changed considerably. There was now an incredible pressure in my lower back and pelvic area. No position I laid in was comfortable, and I couldn't find any method that offered relief. Finally, standing on the side of the bed, leaning over it, breathing, I felt an alarming awareness.

"We need to go to the hospital. Now."

The room went from quiet and peaceful to a bustle of activity. Adam was up and out, getting the car started. My mom-in-law grabbed the birthing ball and headed out, while my mom stayed with me as I monitored what was being taken to the car, remembering the list of things (my type-A ever-present) I wanted to take to the hospital.

Kay had responded by now and was on her way from a nearby town to my house. I spoke with her on the phone as I sat in the car in our driveway. She encouraged that though I was feeling pressure, I was able to talk through my contractions and that was usually unlikely during advanced labor. However, going to the hospital was a good idea and we could always change course depending on how I felt.

I felt we needed to go. She changed direction and headed

on to meet us at the hospital. The hospital ride...that got interesting. It dawned on me on the way to the hospital that I had probably waited too long. It was time to push. The instinct was incredible. It took over.

"Don't get in an accident," I panted, "but get us there, quickly."

Now, fear crashed in. I had waited too long, and now it was time to push. I was in the car, belted into the passenger seat, arching to try and quell the natural instinct to push.

With the fear came a hot, angry adrenaline that completely altered the natural rhythm of my labor. The hurt changed from something natural, smooth and bearable to a choppy, staccato pain that felt angry and disjointed. This new type of pain was jolting. I tensed against it and held my breath.

From the back seat, my mom coached me. "Breathe. Just roll through it. Do not hold your breath."

It was fantastic advice. The only problem was that when I followed her advice, the urge to push was nearly too strong. I did not want to have my baby in the car when the hospital was mere minutes away.

We pulled into the hospital parking lot. I slipped out of the car and stood, leaning over the passenger seat. The fear was beginning to subside, but I was still fighting the natural rhythm of my body.

My good friend appeared. "You're doing great," she said. Her voice was calm.

"I don't think I can do this," I whispered. The idea of waiting to get to the third floor of the hospital and being put in a room before delivering my son seemed like an eternity.

"Yes, you can," she said firmly. "I'm going to apply some counterpressure on your back. You just tell me immediately if you want me to stop or do something else."

Her thumbs expertly pressed against my lower back.

I lost all fight. Down I went, hovering over the pavement. "I *have* to push," I groaned.

The urgency of the situation became apparent to my

friend. Her hands were under my elbows and she tugged me back upright. "Not yet!" she instructed firmly.

"I have to!"

A wheelchair appeared under me. "Get in the wheelchair, Mama," my mother-in-law directed. "We are not having this baby in the parking lot!"

My friend guided me to the wheelchair. I demanded that I had to push.

"Blow candles," she instructed.

"What's that?" I asked.

She demonstrated by blowing small, quick breaths out as though blowing out candles in quick succession. I followed her instructions, and the urge to push became controllable.

My mother-in-law, pushing the wheelchair, barreled through the front doors and to the elevator. She punched the buttons determinedly while my friend leaned over my shoulder, quietly coaching me.

I arched up from the wheelchair to keep from pushing. I knew, beyond a shadow of a doubt, that in a matter of minutes, my baby was going to be here.

My husband was a quiet presence behind me, watching and determined to get us to the maternity wing of the hospital. In a later conversation, he admitted that he was pondering how he was going to "catch" to keep the baby from falling on the elevator floor. My poor mother later told her side of things, where she explained how she dissolved into a puddle of tears as she parked the car, quite certain she was missing the birth.

We pulled up to the desk where nurses awaited us. Some questions were exchanged back and forth—I can't remember exactly what—and I groaned out that my water had broken at 3:00 am, I couldn't time my contractions, and I needed to push—*now.*

They bypassed the triage room and a nurse took me straight into a delivery room across from the nurse's station. Two other nurses were prepping the room. It was apparent that they did not take me seriously once they found out I was having my first child. All work slowed down considerably.

They laid me on the bed, and I twisted over to grip one of the side rails with both hands—it was the only thing I could think to do to not push.

"He's being *born*," I gritted out.

One of the nurses, who stood next to me, typing in information, looked into my face and told me I needed to stay in control. I've never truly wanted to punch someone until that moment. I *somehow* resisted the urge.

Another nurse examined me, and with widened eyes said, "she's full. She's at a ten."

From seemingly out of nowhere, nurses were now buzzing all about me. Where two had been nonchalantly prepping the room, there were now at least seven or eight *quickly* preparing this and that—I honestly don't know what.

All I cared about was the question, "Can I push now?"

The nurse who'd examined me said, "Yes, if you need to push, we will have this baby."

I remember looking down and seeing no one at the end of the bed. Who would catch my baby? I figured if I had to, I would.

The hot, painful fear I felt on the drive was gone. I was back into a normal rhythm of labor. I had regained my confidence. I was in a place where I could have my baby this minute and it would be fine.

My husband, I later learned, had the presence of mind to text my mom and mom-in-law and inform them I was at a "ten." They had been asked to stay out of the room while I was readied for labor. Upon receiving his text, they insisted upon coming into the delivery room. Had it not been for that text and their determined "we're going in there", they'd have missed it all.

Someone asked me about Pitocin, and I said I didn't want any. I heard "Declines Pit!" over the mayhem.

Things are blurry, but sometime within the next minute, the doctor appeared and was scrubbing up, my moms were walking in, and I was in a hospital gown.

I felt uncomfortable lying flat on my back and asked, "can

you please angle the bed up? I don't want to be flat."

Without a word of complaint, the nurses angled my bed up. I could now see over my large, very hard tummy to the doctor's face. I felt much more in control. He calmly gave me brief instructions on how to push.

Upon reflection, I realize now how calm the nurses were when pushing time came. No one was touching me. One nurse came close enough to have me look into her eyes as she repeated the doctor's instructions on pushing, letting me know she was there if I needed help.

I tucked my chin, held my breath, and gave what I *thought* was all I had.

"Is this right?" I grunted.

"No." The doctor's voice was calm and direct. "If you can speak, you're not pushing correctly. Don't talk. Just push."

Including that practice push, my son was born in a total of three pushes.

To put this all into perspective, I arrived at the hospital at somewhere close to 6:10 am, I was checked in at the nurse's desk at 6:20 am, and our son was born at 6:36 am.

Now, I know I told my own birth experience. But there is so much that I gleaned from it, so much that was proven by what happened.

I distinctly remember the change in my labor when I grew truly afraid. And then, I remember the change *back* to my natural rhythm of labor when I was in the hospital and knew I could push and my baby wouldn't land on the floor.

The absence of fear left room for other things. It made room for focus, determination, and excitement. Even though Kai was born so quickly after our arrival and much of the experience is a blur, there was just enough time for me to literally feel the difference between being afraid and letting it go.

No, not every birth experience goes this way. Yes, there will be things I will do differently next time. But I *owned* my birth experience. I stayed in control of it, while releasing control at the same time. It sounds contradictory, but it's not. I stayed in control by being completely in charge of where I gave in. I gave in to my body, to the rhythm, to the discomfort. It was painful, but it was not that hot, angry pain that I felt in the car.

Birth plan, out the window.

Preconceived ideas, out the window.

I held our beautiful son in my arms and felt the most beautiful, powerful emotion in existence. There will never be words to describe it this side of Heaven.

10. THE ADVICE AND SUPPORT CHAPTER

If you feel completely ready and fearless about your labor and delivery, you can skip right on past this chapter.

These are simply some tips and tricks I learned that I'd like to pass on, and since I had my baby in sixteen minutes after check-in, I feel like I might have something someone else may want to hear.

A three-hour labor. A thirty-minute hospital experience.

How in the world did that happen?

Well, a lot of it is genetics. My body is probably programmed to bust a move through labor. Another part of it is pain threshold. I grew up a bit rough and tumble—combine that with severe back pain through my entire third trimester and it's understandable my pain tolerance had been beefed up before labor.

Other factors may have been the weather, the air, the pregnancy, the stock market, the sale on camping tents at the local Wal-Mart. Basically, labor and delivery is not completely explainable. There are no guarantees. My next one could be thirty hours of labor and a three-hour delivery. I certainly hope not, but what if it is?

I'll just do it. I'm a woman, and I can.

However, while so much of labor and delivery feels out of our control, there are some things we *can* control.

The first thing we can do is prep our bodies as best we can. That does not mean you have to be a gym rat or able to fold up like a pretzel. It does not mean you can run ten miles. I do feel, however, that staying active in whatever way you can will help immensely. Giving in and becoming a couch potato will do nothing for you.

At the very end of my pregnancy I could barely swim. I just flopped around until I felt like I accomplished something. Then I laid on my raft feeling rather sassy about myself. I also walked my driveway (about three car lengths) back and forth, back and forth, until I felt my back tell me to stop.

We can also control what we eat. Don't ask for more advice on this from me because I gained forty-five pounds during my pregnancy on a five-foot tall frame, ate strawberry shakes and fish sticks, and my last meal before baby came was fast food. I was proud of myself for eating vegetable quiche and kale chips on the occasion.

Lots of fluids. This one is a biggie. I battled it during my pregnancy. I remember reading and being told I was supposed to drink somewhere between a swimming pool and a small ocean's amount of water every day. I got so tired of flat, plain water. I couldn't do it. So, to get my fluids in, I made sun tea, mellow in flavor and very lightly sweetened. I also would put about three ounces of a tasty juice in a glass and filled the rest with fizzy water. I drank it through a straw and congratulated myself on my water intake.

Rest. It feels easy when you're so tired. But when you're big, big *big* pregnant, getting real rest is a fantasy. The bed is either too soft or too hard. Then it's too hot. So, you crank the air conditioning. Then it's too cold, but no way are you going to turn down the AC, so you uncover half your body. Then that part of you gets chilly but you're too round to reach again and cover back up. Meanwhile, your spouse is lying next to you, shivering. Add the war over the covers and you've got a recipe for zero rest.

I conked out (seriously) while floating on my raft in the pool. It was warm, I was generously swathed in sunscreen, had a floppy hat to cover my face and my fizzy water. No, I don't recommend that for getting adequate rest. I didn't really even mean to fall asleep, but it would happen occasionally.

My Snoogle pillow saved the day. I wrapped it around me, supported my back and put it between my knees. I was able to get reasonable sleep with it. Adam is a cuddle bug by nature. I was an overheated pressure cooker when I was pregnant, so I also creatively used it as a barrier to keep him from smothering me in the night. I remember waking up many times to find he had wiggled his arm completely under the pillow and was snuggling with the entire contraption, including me. I was impressed with the effort and too tired to complain.

Finding ways to rest will be a challenge. Just do your best and go with what's comfortable. That's all I've got for you in that department.

Preparation. I found that as I prepared myself, physically and mentally for labor and delivery, I gained confidence. Because tasks were accomplished and I could check things off my list, my type-A, control freakiness could relax. I felt collected and as put together as one can feel at the end of pregnancy.

I also mentally prepared myself. Want to know how? I didn't spend too much time thinking about labor. I didn't want to think myself out of my own instincts. Yes, of course I wondered and waited, and when Braxton Hicks would happen, I couldn't help speculating at times. But when things didn't pick up and nothing *really* happened, I just let it go.

By the time my labor arrived, I was in a place within myself where I was tapped in. Yes, at times the rest of the world was shut out as I drew further into myself. I took those times to pray, to find peace, and to examine myself. If I found any fear or anxiety, I found ways to deal with it.

I learned by experience that fear will physically impact your birth. It will put you in a state of stress that will stall progress and shatter your natural rhythm. It also hurts a lot more.

Tips I can give for labor? Well, relax. It sounds silly when you're having contractions but it's totally possible. And grind something into your thinking. Contractions are painful. But that pain does not mean something is wrong. It means everything is *right*. Allow yourself to feel it. Breathe through it. Remember that it's passing. Stay in control by letting go.

I remember having to deal with a specific fear. What if something goes wrong and I don't recognize it?

That is probably the deepest fear we'll face during our labor. Having just gone through it and it being so fresh in my mind, I can honestly tell you that I was so involved in laboring that the worries or fears that something could go wrong were out the window. Yes, I made sure I had conquered fear before I reached this point—which certainly helped—but I plain and simply didn't have time to get all worked up about anything else.

Honestly, if you're laboring in some sort of professional setting, my best advice would be to carry on and don't worry about that part. If something goes awry, you're already in the right place. Just focus on yourself. You're the mama. If you've been working at staying in tune with yourself and your baby, you'll just follow that course. Most births happen beautifully.

As far as planning your birth, I would definitely advise you to get a birth plan in place. However, I wouldn't recommend it for the popular reasons. I would say to get a birth plan down on paper to see where *you're* at. Just write it or type it quickly, without thinking too deeply about it. Then, go back over it and read it. You may be surprised at what you've written. It may be very telling about your ideas and wishes. An even better idea is to type up a specific labor plan, detailing how you want to labor at home, how you want the environment around you, and who you want nearby.

I had decided I was going to give birth as naturally as I possibly could. That meant, for me, that I wanted no medications or interventions unless it was absolutely necessary. Well, I also had to decide, as far as the Epidural is concerned, what "absolutely necessary" meant. My decision was that I trusted myself enough to know if I needed it when the time came. Pretty simple, I know, but the simplicity took the stress out of it for me.

I had one friend who gave birth to both of her children without an Epidural tell me that she prepared by imagining the pain was going to be the worst possible pain there is to feel in this world. She expected that, prepared for that, and when labor finally came, it wasn't as painful as she expected. The pleasant surprise of it made her able to cope with the contractions.

I found that rather creative and unconventional. I decided I'd try it. I nearly didn't get to the hospital in time, waiting for that major pain. I'm not saying that's the best way to go about it, but you can find little ways in your mind to get on your mark, ready and set. You know you.

If there's one thing I can share here, it's to be completely and totally sure that your decisions are coming from the inside of *you*, and not from outside influences. There is no other human being on this earth that should have the ability to tell you how you're going to labor and what you're going to do. Trusted sources may have things they'd like to share with you, but *you're* putting in the work. You have ultimate veto power.

When you have that confidence, you can change your mind in the middle of whatever is going on without a sense of guilt riding you. The last thing in the world you should have to worry about is disappointing someone else because you made a decision they may not agree with.

If you've decided you want to have an unmedicated birth but are afraid you won't be able to follow through when the time comes, I just want you to know something.

You can do it.

Don't kid yourself. It's painful. It's uncomfortable. But it's not the end of the world. Don't associate your pain with an injury or wound. You're not injured, you're not wounded. Your body is doing exactly what it's supposed to do. Buff up in your mind, flex those muscles, and then relax all the others in your body.

Also realize that your body is going to do its thing. If your mind is saying "Wait—I didn't tell you to do this. I'm not okay with this," you're going to go to battle against yourself. That's the perfect environment for fear to grow. Allow your mind to be open, to realize your body is instinctively doing what it's supposed to do and learn to go with it. Stay in control by letting go.

If you start to move into a position to handle the pain without thinking about it, move into that position. I found myself rocking back and forth across my birthing ball, and my mind and breathing followed that rhythm. My body was then in sync and managing the pain was so much easier. The music, dim lights, and the calm around me allowed me to do whatever I needed to do. There is no right or wrong way to move during labor.

You are powerful. You are carrying your baby, and your body is equipped with everything it needs to accomplish the task. Buy in to that belief. Close the door on fear. It's unnecessary. Forget about what others may think or your idea of how you should look or act during labor. Trust me, we are all admiring you.

Focus on that sweet baby, let your mind become so engaged with that little one inside you that every heartbeat is dedicated to him or her.

And then go with your gut.

11. THE REFLECTION CHAPTER

Not every birth experience is going to go the same way. They're as different as fingerprints.

Not every birth experience is perfectly smooth, either. Mine sure didn't feel smooth when I was in the car, groaning in fright and trying to keep my son from being born in the car.

That doesn't mean success or failure, either. I think that, above everything else during my pregnancy and childbirth experience, I learned to just trust myself. I learned to allow myself to be a woman. We tend to be *way* too hard on ourselves and become frightened when things start to happen that don't fit our plans.

We're bigger than that. We are strong enough to stay in control of fear, despite the changes. And, when fear comes against us, we are strong enough to press on anyway. Fear battles over our minds at the most vulnerable times. It rushed in on me during that precarious drive to the hospital. But even in the midst of my labor, I was reminded that I could fight it.

I remember seeing a woman I knew in the store when Kai was several weeks old. The woman's pregnant daughter-in-law was with her. They beamed over the baby, and then began talking about the girl's own pregnancy. It became apparent she was quite fearful of what was to come.

Something came over me and I looked into the girl's eyes and said, "you can do this. Your body is incredible, and you are perfectly capable. You're going to do a great job."

The girl blinked at me in surprise, and I watched her eyes fill with tears. That she doubted herself was clearly obvious. I continued to affirm her until I saw the shadow of fear diminish.

I remember all too well the horror stories people felt inclined to share about risky birth experiences, tragic outcomes, etc. People are often utterly tactless when it comes to sharing stories with pregnant women.

I began to combat that by responding with, "I'm not going to allow myself to think that way. I'm fighting for a smooth labor and delivery for my baby."

People reacted to my determination with surprise, confusion, some doubt, and even some laughter. It was appalling. What is it in us that makes us cling to the negative, to spread fear? Why do we enjoy causing reactions in others that aren't positive?

Even mothers who had been through labor and delivery shared scary stories they'd heard or experienced. Why is this? Is it because they felt insecure and afraid, and therefore passed it on?

I'll never know or understand all the reasons. All I can say is that it does *not* have to feel that way! You can have a pregnancy, even a bumpy one, without being overtaken by fear. In fact, fear will cause more bumps in the road and we don't have to go about it that way.

Books that relay their passion due to sad experiences may defeat their own purposes. Mindsets that are meant to be empowering can cause doubt and fear when going down a road of suspicion.

We need to defeat this thinking in our culture. We need to make it a *must* to believe in one another's abilities, to encourage one another. Instead of trying to persuade one another *how* to go about birth, why not affirm one another that we *can* go about birth, and then support the road we each choose to take?

12. THE <u>YOU</u> CHAPTER

You, amazing mama, are pregnant. You are carrying your precious little one. You are making choices that you feel are best for you and your child. These choices, made free of fear and doubt, are steps that you take toward making your little miracle happen.

That is powerful. That is incredible. And you are completely capable.

Your journey is underway. You will be a mom. You will be an *amazing* mom. You have been given instincts specific to bringing a child into the world and then caring for that child. There is a love inside of you that is incomparable. Your baby can feel that and will feel it from now on.

No one will be able to cuddle your little one like you can. No one will be able to comfort them when they're sick like you can. The nurturer in you is irreplaceable and second to none.

You have made it to this point—look how far you've come!

Your labor will arrive, and you will know *now is the time.*

Your breathing will start, every instinct in your body will ramp up several gears. Your every thought and focus will be about your own body and the baby within. Your focus will shift between your baby and you, and that is because there are times when you will need to focus entirely on what you're doing as you bring you baby into this world. You will turn inside yourself. You will be so utterly *connected* to yourself, your body and your instincts, that you will take a journey no one—not even those standing beside you—will take.

You'll feel discomfort and pain. You'll feel pressure.

You will work toward your goal, you will be wherever you are, and you will give birth. You will know that you're not perfect. Not everything will go exactly the way you expected—it never does. But you're strong enough to carry on anyway.

You'll cry. You'll groan. You'll sweat.

But you'll do it. You understand that this is apart of this miraculous journey. It's not an injury. It's not a wound. It's not a misfire or malfunction. It's the process. And it's painfully beautiful.

No one else can say they brought your child into the world. It's something that you did. No matter what happens or how your birth goes, you should know that you are absolutely, without a doubt, incredible.

You are instinctively *mom.*

You didn't need another book telling you which vitamins to take and which foods to avoid. You didn't need more statistics on interventions, immunizations, etc. There are books and apps *galore* for that.

You needed a book that was about *you*, the *heart* of you. You needed affirmation and encouragement. You needed to see that this is something that does not need to be overly complicated, this is something beautiful and wonderful and something we as women just *do*. You needed to know that there isn't just one trail of steps for you to walk in. There is a path made up of millions and millions of women all throughout time, that you are walking this path but taking *your own steps,* and this is your freedom and your right.

You needed something you could read, close the cover and, with a sigh, say, "I can do this."

And then, you will hold your baby in your arms, and you will rejoice in your victory.

You did it.

www.ingramcontent.com/pod-product-compliance
Lightning Source LLC
Chambersburg PA
CBHW051414250726
48655CB00003B/1050